I0414011

Kettlebells Exercise:

An Ultimate Guide To Kettlebells Exercise.

Text Copyright © Alicia Labert

All rights reserved. No part of this guide may be reproduced in any form without permission in writing from the publisher except in the case of brief quotations embodied in critical articles or reviews.

Legal & Disclaimer

The information contained in this book and its contents is not designed to replace or take the place of any form of medical or professional advice; and is not meant to replace the need for independent medical, financial, legal or other professional advice or services, as may be required. The content and information in this book has been provided for educational and entertainment purposes only.

The content and information contained in this book has been compiled from sources deemed reliable, and it is accurate to the best of the Author's knowledge, information and belief. However, the Author cannot guarantee its accuracy and validity and cannot be held liable for any errors and/or omissions. Further, changes are periodically made to this book as and when needed. Where appropriate and/or necessary, you must consult a professional (including but not limited to your doctor, attorney, financial advisor or such other professional advisor) before using any of the suggested remedies, techniques, or information in this book.

Upon using the contents and information contained in this book, you agree to hold harmless the Author from and against any damages, costs, and expenses, including any legal fees potentially resulting from the application of any of the information provided by this book. This disclaimer applies to any loss, damages or injury caused by the use and application, whether directly or indirectly, of any advice or information presented, whether for breach of contract, tort, negligence, personal injury, criminal intent, or under any other cause of action.

You agree to accept all risks of using the information presented inside this book.

You agree that by continuing to read this book, where appropriate and/or necessary, you shall consult a professional (including but not limited to your doctor, attorney, or financial advisor or such other advisor as needed) before using any of the suggested remedies, techniques, or information in this book.

Table of Contents

Introduction

Kettlebells or girya is a traditional cast iron weights that are used for ballistic exercises. Their physical appearance resembles that of a cannon ball with a looped handle. They look small bawling balls with a large handle on the top.

Russian lifters have had kettlebells as their weapon of choice for over a century now. They are so popular in Russia that all weight lifters and strongmen are referred to as kettlebell men. It is fascinating to know that it is now that they are making their way into the American markets. The surge in their popularity in the last one decade can be attributed to their three cardinal functions. They combine cardiovascular development building strength and enhancing flexibility. They are designed in such a way that the weight hangs just a few inches off the handle making it a little more difficult to control. The weights offer everything a dumbbell does and in addition, their super thick handles challenge your grip making your core work extra hard burning calories in effect.

Chapter 1: Kettlebells Exercise

Kettlebells versatility makes them ideal for vigorous exercises that involve major muscles and in the process burning fat and building power. With kettlebells, one no longer needs to spend hours in the gym as an excellent kettlebell workout takes only 15 minutes three times a week to get the same results as with a dumbbell. This makes them an ideal training program for both men and women looking for the best results in the shortest time possible.

Kettlebells gain in popularity can also be attributed to the fact that it focuses around three core lifts- the swing, the snatch, the clean and the jerk. All these concentrate the muscle to work as a group. In the process, every single muscle is worked hard strengthening your core and building core stability. The entire body is worked in less time compared to other forms of exercise.

Benefits Of Using Kettlebells

Building lean muscle

The dynamic of kettlebell training provides the opportunity for building lean muscle, and condition the cardiovascular system. Most people forget the importance of building lean muscle when trying to get in shape. The lean muscle does not just make the body look nice but also play a key role in metabolism and energy levels helping the body burn fat.

Versatile resistance training

The versatility provided by kettlebells beats about all other kinds of training options out there. They are not only more convenient than weights and machines which use more time in terms of trips to the gym. The design of the kettlebell is in such a way that they use more muscle groups to keep the weight controlled. They work the muscles from all angles encouraging well strength building and increasing flexibility. Weightlifters, professional athletes, law enforcement officers all use kettlebells to get the resistance that helps them build strength and agility required in their profession.

Cardiovascular training

Thorough cardiovascular training is vital in all kinds of training. It helps the cardiovascular system to effectively and efficiently distribute blood and oxygen to all body parts especially the muscles and brain. The body is, therefore able to use its strength and increase the brain's ability to focus more and for longer periods. The dynamic of kettlebell routine can be done in conjunction with strength training making it more efficient within a short time.

Building self-confidence

One of the most important benefits of kettlebell training is building self-confidence in the individual. It gives more confidence to feel stronger, more flexible, be more agile and feel fit. The physical benefits of working out improve self-esteem giving the trainee more emotional energy.

Convenience

The most attractive attribute of the kettlebell is the convenience in which they allow one to train. There are very few workout programs that allow one to work out all muscles of the body in conjunction with cardiovascular training without necessarily having to go to the gym. The good thing is that the training only takes about 20 minutes three times a week. Training with kettlebells requires only a few sets of kettlebells and a training program fit for your body type and aspirations.

Portable

Unlike barbells and other training exercise equipment kettlebells are portable hence no need to miss a workout. One can even carry a couple of kettlebells when out of town or on holiday.

Full body workout

Kettlebells provide full body workout, the swigs, squats, snatches, lunges, deadlifts, and presses are all compound exercises that work on all muscle groups. This makes little exercise very effective saving time and energy.

Breaks monotony

If you have been training using machines and dumbbells and hit a plateau where you are no longer able to gain size or progress to heavier weights then switching to the kettlebell based regime will shock the system into new growth not to mention its fun. This breaks the monotony of the gym and also acts as a change of scenery.

Cheap

To get into great shape one only needs at least a pair or two of kettlebells to build functional fitness. Kettlebells are generally cheap going for about 2-3 dollars per kilogram. The money spent on kettlebells is money well spent as you will not find such value for money as in gym membership or overpriced prices for other excise equipment.

Improve coordination

When you are swinging and passing the kettlebell around, your brain and muscles must coordinate effectively in order to perform the necessary movements. This increases your hand and eye coordination and the increased coordination will transfer to all the other associated activities.

Correct imbalances

If you are used to training using machines and barbells you will find that you have a stronger side that will compensate for the weaker side when necessary. Kettlebells swiftly identify and corrects the imbalances through dingle limb exercises.

Time saving

Many individuals dismiss working out due to time constraints as they are busy with other stuff but a set of portable kettlebells eliminates this excuse as it only requires about 15-20 minutes for an intense workout plan. Majority of kettlebell workouts are short and intense. If you find yourself taking substantially longer, then it maybe time to increase your intensity and reduce your rest period.

Developing massive power

Olympic lifts such as the clean & jerk and snatch when performed, increases explosive power and places a new spin on these exercises as compared to performing them with a barbell or dumbbell.

Improves flexibility

Kettlebell exercises work on postural muscles in such a manner that they increase flexibility hence better posture for the trainee.

Chapter 2: Types Of Kettlebells

There are different types of kettlebells. The most popular types are powder coat kettlebell, cast iron kettlebell, and steel competition kettlebell

Powder coat kettlebell

The difference between powder cast kettlebell and cast iron kettlebell is the powder coating which makes it more durable. The colored bands on the handles indicate weight.

Cast iron kettlebell

They are commonly used for muscle building. They have thick smooth handles optimized to prevent chafing. They have a flat base for easy storage. The kettlebells are stamped in kilograms and their sizes depend on weight. Exercising using these kettlebells, depend on an individual and how much one wants to challenge the shoulders.

Steel competition kettlebells

They are all of the same sizes regardless of weight hence any weight will always fit in your hands in the same exact way. They are color coded to international standards.

Rubber coated kettlebells as their name suggests are coated with rubber and do not undergo rust.they also don't scratch. They come in different sizes depending on weight.

Vinyl kettlebells are coated with vinyl a synthetic resin comprising of different colors that give it a sophisticated appeal.

Classic kettlebells increase in size as the corresponding weight increases. A 50kg kettlebell is bigger than a 10 kg kettlebell.

Lifting Techniques

The following techniques detail the correct form and how to go about common kettlebell exercises. If you are new to kettlebell training it is recommended that you get a partner or coach who is familiar with the exercises as an incorrect form can lead to back pains. This happens when there is an intense amount of stress placed on the posterior chain when doing the swings. Working with kettlebells requires a combination of proper form and an understanding of the correct posture, grip balance, and transitions. Just like with other exercises equipment it is important to learn how to correctly use the kettlebells to avoid injuries and to ensure a successful workout plan. There are excellent DVDs available to help train one with the proper handling techniques of kettlebells but one would still need to work with a certified instructor in order to get the right moves and perform them safely.

Style

There are three different styles of lifting kettlebell which all bring slightly different results.

1. Hard style. This is said to be the original kettlebell workout and involves generating explosive power and strength. Kime technique is the principle behind hard style and is an all-out effort in every repetition. The aim is to produce the power needed to swing, snatch, press or squat but increasing power is key. This style utilizes fast rigid movements as opposed to smooth and fluid motions. For this reason, it is also called the Russian kettlebell challenge. Hard styles maximize both extremes in terms of tension and strength while still concentrating on relaxation and speed. The tenser the muscle the more the force produced. They increase strength by contacting muscles harder. Each workout produces more output but in less time.
2. Sports style. This style combines power and strength for overall endurance. It requires an athlete to work under a sub maximal load, lifting the kettlebell as many times as possible in a set time frame of ten minutes.
3. Juggling. It is insane to conceptualize the idea of one juggling a steel ball weighing 10 or20 pounds but it has already become a very popular style of kettlebell lifting. It provides increased ability in core strength and resistance to rotation. It also enhances hand-eye coordination and brings powerful pulling strength and above all its fun.

HOLDS

A kettlebell can be held in different ways to achieve a range of the required results. The way you hold, grip, grab and the angle determines the muscle to be used and the difficulty to be endured. Using one hand or both during a workout also affects the result.

- Racked. In this position, the arm is bent with the upper arm held tight to the body and the hand in line with the chin. The handle is in your palm and the bell is on the outside.
- By the horns. This is a common position for beginners and involves holding the kettlebell by the horns. The bell is held close to the chest.
- Squeeze or crush. This is almost similar to by the horns but instead of gripping by the horns you hold the bell by squeezing it with the base of your fingers. The lack of grip makes it necessary for the arm muscles to compensate.
- Waiter. The kettlebell is made to rest in your open palm.

POSTURE

When exercising with kettlebell it is very important to maintain the appropriate posture so as to prevent injury. Primary consideration should be made to avoid hunching forward with rounded shoulders. The head should face forward with the eyes focused roughly 6 feet ahead down. The spine should retain its natural S curve. This position makes you look like you are just about to sit down on a chair. In this position, you should be able to place a stick along your spine from your head to your hips with contacts with the head shoulders and upper glutes.

Chapter 3: Warm Up And Cool Down

Warm up and cool down

Warming up is very important before starting any excise and kettlebell training is no exception to this. One should warm up correctly to avoid muscle injuries. Mobility is key in any workout. Keeping your joints mobile ensures movement without compensation while reducing the chances of getting injured. This keeps your joints strong and healthy. A good warm-up program should not only ready you physically but also mentally and neurologically because the body needs to be turned on ready for action.

The joints to focus on include

- Neck – cervical spine
- Shoulders – both shoulder capsule and girdle
- Upper back – thoracic spine
- Wrist and elbows
- Upper pelvis
- Lower pelvis
- Knees and ankles

While many of the warm-up activities offer circulation mobility and joint preparation they focus mainly on the engagement required to move a kettlebell effectively and efficiently.

Around the world

This is done by picking the kettlebell and swinging it around your waistline. You should prioritize moving the kettlebell smoothly and ensure your midline is solid. Undertake this exercise with a light weight so as to achieve smooth movement of the bell through space while maintaining control.

Make sure you maintain a circular kettlebell path and avoid swinging it low across front and back. The midline should be stable with minimal deviation from the vertical standing position. The exercise should be about developing control and mastery of moving the kettlebell through space. Do not shift your weight to accommodate the path of the kettlebell. The kettlebell should never lose its path as it passes from hand to hand. Since your body is intelligent enough to choose the direction that feels more natural and easy you should always try to balance between your dominant and no dominant sides.

Figure eight

This requires a stable and static body and the only movements is that of the arms and the kettlebell. This move warms your legs and hip hinge. You begin in a wide stance and smoothly pass the kettlebell between your legs and around one and back again around the other leg drawing a figure eight.

Halos

It allows one to move and control the kettlebell while maintaining a strong and stable midline. It offers a complete

Chapter 4: Nutrition

It would be unwise to assert that nutrition is a one size fits all kind of gambit. Some rules must be followed to ensure your body transformation. One should ensure they are getting enough proteins without exceeding on calories. Macronutrients are vital. For a fit and healthy body your body requires the right nutrients and in the correct proportions. Most people take the wrong route when they decide to diet, they do this by lowering their caloric intake and this involves cutting down on carbohydrates. This would be correct if the carbs come from junk food cakes excess bread and candy. When the body is exposed to drastic changes in the diet it adapts to chemical processes as it aims to safeguard its glucose stores.

Carbohydrates are the main source of energy that fuels the functioning of the muscles. Carbohydrates are broken down in the body into smaller elements that the body can utilize. They are stored in form of glycogen in muscles fat and liver and can be accessed when the need arises. For this reason, sudden drastic changes can be counter-productive because if the body noticed a drop in supply it would adjust by protecting the already available. This means metabolism slows down to preserve energy. During extreme carbohydrate shortage when glycogen stores are depleted the body metabolizes its own protein to provide energy. This leads to the breakdown of muscle skin hair and bones making the body have that appearance of a starving person.

Apart from providing energy needed for cellular function and growth carbohydrates also perform the following functions within the body;

- Regulate blood sugar levels
- Help in calcium absorption
- Provide nutrients for probiotics in the intestinal tract
- Assist in regulating blood pressure and cholesterol levels
- Fuel the CNS and the brain

In maintaining a healthy diet selecting protein, vitamins and minerals from natural sources while at the same time avoiding processed foods serves as the most important step towards maintaining health.

An appropriate diet consists of the following elements;

- Proteins from fish lean meats and nuts
- Vegetables and fruits
- While grains and alternate carbs such as barley corn meal and beans
- Dairy including milk cheese and yoghurt
- Healthy fats and oils

- Limited amounts of refined grains eg potatoes and white rice
- Minimal amounts of other items like salt sugar and alcohol.

There is no ideal diet plan that will fit the needs of every individual and when planning your diet common sense and some little knowledge regarding ingredients and nutrients is important. Always consider the following

- Pay attention to the size of the portions. One should eat better and not more
- Select a wide range of food sources that will help cover your nutritional needs
- At each meal the choice of carbs to be taken should be carefully chosen
- Always choose foods that are of higher quality. Less processed, more natural
- Always take breakfast, and healthy snacks in midmorning and mid afternoon
- Ensure you include a small portion of lean protein
- Avoid caffeine and drink green tea
- Never underestimate the need to stay hydrated. Drink plenty of water.
- Add spices and herbs to help aid digestion

When working out itys important to keep the body hydrated to replace the fluids lost through sweats. Intense workouts can create a huge water demand of even 2-3 gallons of water daily. Water is important for the following functions

- Provides the fluid portion of blood that transports oxygen and other nutrients.
- Gets rid of toxins and cellular waste products from the body in solution form
- Helps in thermoregulation
- Helps improve digestion

Chapter Five: Work Outs

When you are new to kettlebell work outs or you are currently out of shape and you want to ease out into routine work out slowly its necessary to start out slow with the basics. There is no need to go to complex intense movements when you are still learning and increasing your body conditioning. Start slowly and move on when you feel you need additional challenge. When planning your work out regime don't forget the legs. You can work on the legs by doing the kettlebell suitcase squats or kettlebell lunges. Suitcase squats are easier and simple because they require no skill but you will need two bells. When doing the lunges you will need to rack the kettlebell in the crook of your arm giving you the perfect excuse to learn how to do the kettlebell clean

Kettlebell exercises are space saving compared to other exercises like the treadmill or even a gym. Unlike other weights and techniques kettlebells variations and techniques are just endless. The workouts are not meant for men only but can also be done by women. Women who complain of trouble trying control weight loss because of slow metabolism can undertake kettlebell swings to shed those unwanted pounds.

Kettlebell swing ids the fundamental exercise as the movement is the foundation upon which most beginners work outs are built. They build up you muscle endurance while gently easing your body into an exercise habit. Including swings in your workout routine makes you strong and fit to move on to more complex and demanding kettlebell moves.

Exercises involving the upper body can be divided into two i.e. push and pull. By pushing you work your body on the chest shoulders and triceps and by pulling you work your upper back and biceps. Failure to include push and pull in your work out leads to unbalance and may lead to injuries.

CORE WORK OUTS

This workout exercises your whole body. The core mostly feels the burn when you done. The exercises are perfect in that they improve core strength by enhancing the strength and flexibility of all related muscles extending outwards to the extremities. The shape and movement of the kettlebells at the end of your arms keeps you off balance and more muscles are required to stabilize your body. The fact that the kettlebell is not stationary in your hands adds to the dynamics of each movement, forcing muscles to compensate for the changing centre of gravity.

KETTLEBELL ARMS

To completely work out the arms one needs to work out all the muscle groups which include the biceps triceps and forearm. Depending on the intended aim one can use heavy weights to build muscle and strength with lower reps or can do more exercises with more repetitions when burning fats is the aim

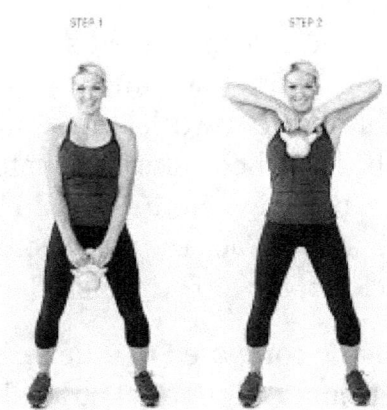

KETTLEBELL PRESS

The kettlebell press or overhead press is a wonderful strength building lift for all pressing needs. It is unlike a normal dumbbell press or dumbbell because of the offset nature of the kettlebell. If it's your first time then you in for a big surprise. The awkward shape of the kettlebell makes it handling a little more complex as it requires the participant have some technique if he is to handle it with some degree of control. By having the weight rest against the back of your arm it tries to pull you out of your groove and into a somehow dangerous position. One needs to learn how to clean and rack the bell first and then follow it up with pressing. Clean and racks are a prerequisite position before executing the military press or other lifts. A solid and consistent clean makes the press successful. It does not matter how strong you are if your clean delivers the weight to a poor rack then the pres will be a struggle. Breath is an important aspect of creating tension and relaxation. Prepare your body for the impact which should be minimal.

How it's done

This part of the lift essentially gets the bell to a racked position at your chest with your arm at rest against your body. Your fist should be below your chin and your legs locked out feet set slightly wider than shoulder width distance apart in length. To hold the bell correctly at the rack, you will have to lock your hips and knees by clenching your glutes and tightening your quads.

Execution

1. Clean a kettlebell to your shoulder by extending through the legs and hip as you pull the kettlebell towards your shoulder. As you doing that rotate your wrist so that your palm faces inward. This is the starting position.
2. Look at the kettlebell as you press it up and out overhead.
3. Slowly lower the kettlebell to your shoulders and repeat. For maximum stability ensure you contact your lat butt and stomach.

When in this position you will be forcing your hips forward creating space for your arms to rest against your body while the bell is on the rack.

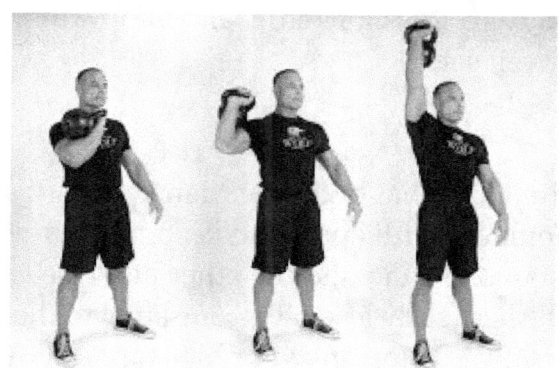

KETTLEBELL SWING

This is a classic kettlebell movement and is perfect for beginners. It is a fundamental movement for a great group of kettlebell movements. The muscles targeted include hips, legs, glutes, back and shoulders. The swing utilizes a hip thrust important to other movements such as the one arm snatch. To develop maximum fitness strength and endurance levels one needs to learn effective and efficient swing techniques.

You need to find a kettlebell you can confidently swing and place it on the floor between your feet. Start with the kettlebell slightly in front of you positioned between your legs which should be wider than shoulder width. Look straight ahead and keep your neck in a neutral position with your knees slightly bent, your back flat and hip pointing backwards. Do not go too low as this should be between a squat and a stand. Hike the kettlebell behind you like in American football but keep hold of the kettlebell stretching the hamstrings. Count to three in your head and then fluidly and in one continuous motion extend your hips forcefully and extend the kettlebell along its arc till it reaches about the chest length. Contract your abs and glutes for stability. In this movement your arms act as just a hook and the power originates from movement of the hips and the posterior chain i.e. glutes lower back and hamstrings. This movement should be fluid with no rest in between reps. the important part in this exercise is to work with the swinging motion rather than against it.

Swinging the kettlebells higher than chest height is not efficient and there's little to be gained. You breathe out at the apex of the swing. You can target your abs by focusing on tilting your pelvis up at the top of the swing.

As you let the kettlebell fall free back between your legs breathe in hold your breath. The hips should move backwards to allow loading of the posterior chain to enable power for the subsequent swing.

Single arm kettlebell swing

This works in the same way as a Russian kettlebell but now in unilateral fashion. You alternate the arms in between sets.

Execution

The starting position is similar to that of the Russian kettlebell swing. You need to stand straight with your feet shoulder width apart and keeping your neck in a neutral position. With the kettlebell handle in one hand and the other hand free to swing and drive momentum, bend your knees slightly lowering your body to the ground and driving your hips backwards. Explode upwards moving your hips forwards and contracting your abs and glutes for stability. Swing the kettlebell until your arms is parallel to the floor. Your other arm swings to aid in momentum. Lower the kettlebell to the staring position. Do not switch the arms between each rep but rather wait till the end to ensure muscles work to their full potential.

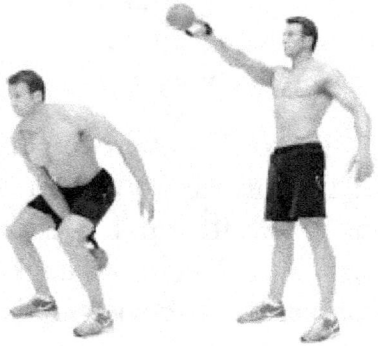

One arm kettlebell swing

This is a great movement as it engages the back and legs. It takes some time to get it right so one should take it slow in the beginning. The muscles involved include the back, legs, glutes and core.

Execution

Start with legs shoulder width apart and place the kettlebell between your feet. Hold the kettlebell in one hand with a loose grip and your thumb pointing behind you to prevent the kettlebell from hitting your wrist. Pull the bell up to your shoulder level and in the process exhale and tense the muscles in your core and glutes. The aim is to keep the kettlebell close to your body at all times. Refrain from swinging the arm not lifting the bell at all times and keep it tight. In a slow but controlled motion return the kettlebell back to the starting position. Do not switch arms between reps but swap between sets instead. It is also important to engage your core at the top of the movement.

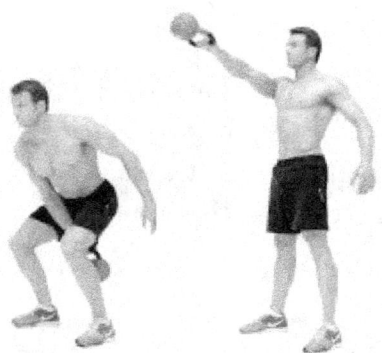

Kettlebell deadlift

This is the king of all leg movements. The muscles targeted include legs arms back core and glutes.

Execution

In this routine stand with your legs a little closer than your shoulder width and place the kettlebell in between your legs. Squat down and hold the kettlebell with both hands in such a way that your knuckles point in front of you. Your knees and hip should be bent and your back flat. Tighten your arms and keep them extended while engaging your core and glutes. Slowly stand up driving your hips upwards and pause at the top to squeeze before reversing the movement and putting the kettlebell to the starting postion. Don't overextend and roll backwards. The reps should be smooth instead of a fast one.

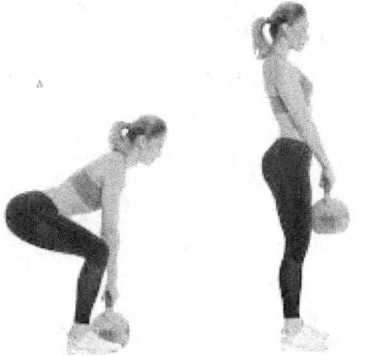

KETTLEBELL ARM WORK OUT

When using kettlebells to work on arms, the shape and grip will influence the target muscle. You can target your triceps and biceps differently. Depending on the aim of the work out you can use heavier weights in case you want to build muscles and strength with lower reps or you can do more exercises with more repetitions if you want to burn some calories. A complete training should work on all the groups of muscles which are biceps triceps and forearm.

KETTLEBELL ROWS

This is a wonderful variation from the traditional bent over row. This exercise primarily works on the muscles of the back. It also works on the legs core and hips. There are different ways of doing it but in all the variations you should always push your butt behind you as much as possible to begin the movement.

ONE ARM KETTELBELL

By making a staggered stance the kettlebell will go next to your front foot. Move the elbow up towards the ceiling. The elbow should be close to the body. Slowly bring the bell up to near your stomach.

TWO ARM KETTLEBELL ROW

This movement is great for working the back and shoulders. It depends on a straight Back and tight core. The muscles targeted are arms back and shoulders.

Execution

Stand with feet at shoulder width apart and place a kettlebell in front of each foot. While keeping your back flat and your neck in a neutral position slightly bend at the knees. Grab both kettlebells and pull them towards your stomach while still avoiding standing up or moving your knees and back. The movement resembles that of a rowing machine with your elbows moving backwards. The movement in both arms should be equal to each other. This move should be fluid while also keeping the elbows close to the body. Tense your core at the top of the rep and keep everything tight then slowly lower the weights in a controlled motion back to the starting position.

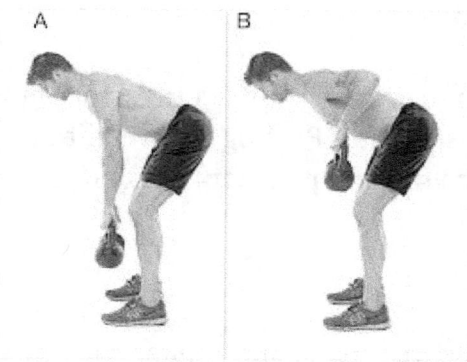

The renegade alternating kettlebell

This variation incorporates a whole lot of additional muscle groups. You assume a push up position and hold each kettlebell with one hand. You then shift the weight to one kettlebell while you do a row with the other.

KETTLEBELL RUSSIAN TWIST

This is one of the most effective methods of building a strong and defined abs and core strength. The muscles targeted are the abs and oblique's.

Execution

The starting position looks similar to that of a crunch but now with the legs about a hip apart. With your feet flat on the ground sit with the legs bent at the knees. With both hands pick up the kettlebell and bring it to your chest. Lean back a little bit to make a 45- degree angle. Now twist your torso from left to right starting at the waist. Do not swing the weight but rather pick it from your left side and bring it over your body and place it on the other side and then repeat. Always ensure you keep the movement in control.

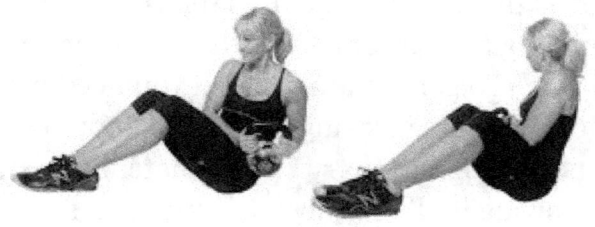

KETTLEBELL SQUAT

Kettlebell squat is a superior exercise for an average person who doesn't have good flexibility mobility and core strength. Placing the weight in front of the body makes it easier on the spine and knees making it easier to stay in the best position as compared to traditional barbell back squat.

Execution

> Sit back like you are seated in a chair, adjust you back to stay flat as your spine is lengthened and chest stays tall. The foot position should be narrower stance than normal mostly between shoulder and hip width apart. Perfect the move before plunging into your regular workouts. The work out is done at the beginning of your routine with sub maximal weight to achieve a nice warm up. This exercise is superior to other forms of squat so take your time to learn the move properly and you will be glad you did it.
> This workout takes it easy on you with only two different exercises. Make sure you pick a kettlebell that you can handle comfortably. Do each exercise for 50-40-30-20-10 reps.

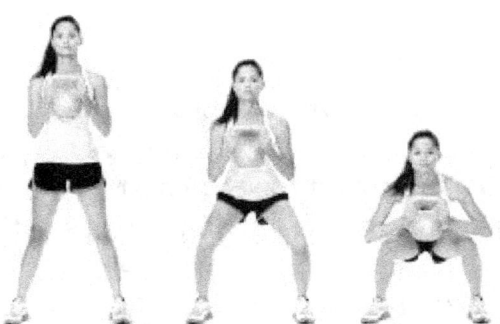

KETTLEBELL SNATCH

This combines the kettlebell press and swing. It is referred to as the czar by some Russians. It is vital in building a superior core with hip power and shoulder strength to produce unbelievable power. To perform the snatch you need first to have learnt to do the swing so that you know your arc of swing. The key is to know your shoulder mobility and flexibility before you can progress to trying the snatch. You start with the kettlebell in between your legs. You swing it all the way back and then swing it back all the way so that your arm is directly above your head. The repeated swings up and down will burn off some calories and build the muscles affected by the press and swing target. Ensure the bell does not bhang your arm when performing this as that would mean you either using too much weight, your technique is poor or the arc of your swing is too wide. Apart from posterior chain conditioning the snatch is also a brilliant exercise for the shoulder girdle. For this move you need to quickly decentralize and stabilize the kettlebell and this builds incredible strength and stability. For many persons with weak posterior muscles and conditioning the snatch acts as powerful remedy with a powerful hip hinge. The overhead position has to be stable with no deviation. This is important in developing shoulder stability.

Another great benefit of snatch is that it can be great alternative to the overhead press if you have shoulder issues particularly if you have been working out with barbell press. Kettlebell snatch is magnificent in developing aerobic capacity. It is impactful as compared to many other activities and has impressive metabolic response making it an alternative to traditional aerobic activities.

Since the kettlebell snatch strengthens stabilizes and builds the aerobic capacity it is referred to as the mother of all kettlebell exercises due to the multitude of benefits it brings.

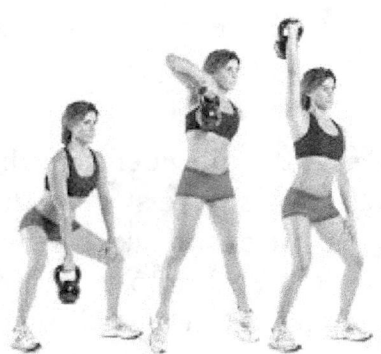

KETTLEBELL LUNGES

The muscles targeted are the quadriceps, glutes, hamstrings and calf muscles. The core is activated due to the unilateral movement required of this exercise. The kettlebells are held for an extended period of time to help build forearms and traps. Lunges are useful for sports requiring frequent lunging activities eg tennis badminton fencing and even soccer and basketball.

Execution

Step forward with your right foot and assume a lunge position. When in this position pass the kettlebell through your legs to your other hand and then stand up straight. Step forward with your left foot and repeat the steps again as many times as needed.

Backward stepping lunge is one of the easiest methods to learn the lunge and get used to the balance. It allows you to control the pressure on your knees completely hence good for those with tricky knees.

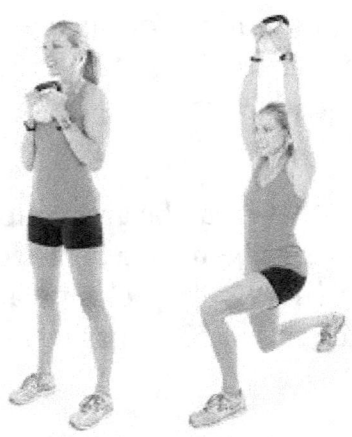

KETTLEBELL HIGH PULL

This exercise works on the upper body. The movement starts at the heels rising through the hips. The muscles targeted are the arms, shoulders, traps, legs and glutes.

 Execution

You start the exercise by standing a little bit wider than shoulder width apart and the feet angled at 45 degrees. The kettlebell should start on the ground between you legs. While keeping your core tight squat down and take the kettlebell handle in one hand. Move up with your hips and push your heels into the ground. Move into a standing position while at the same time pulling the kettlebells upwards. The elbows drive the kettlebells upwards and once at the top hold momentarily before going back to the starting position. During this execise ensure your chest is high and your core is tight throughout the movement. This aids in stability and control. The kettlebell should start on the ground and return there after every complete rep.

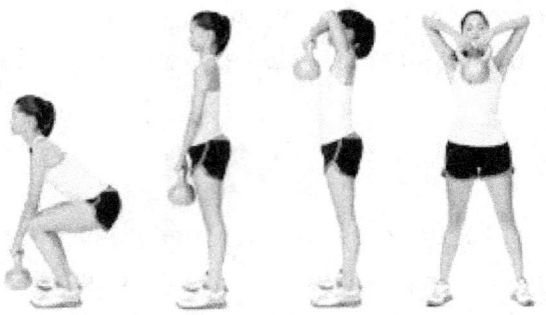

Conclusion

Kettlebell is an effective way of working out as it is a fun and dynamic way of improving your overall fitness. It also assists in weight loss. The workouts are easy to do whether at home, at the gym or at training centre. For a well toned body and weight maintenance the kettlebells provide a fun and quick way to exercise and achieve the body you desire.

When undertaking the work outs, it's important to follow the safety advice and precautions indicated to avoid possible injuries.

www.ingramcontent.com/pod-product-compliance
Lightning Source LLC
Chambersburg PA
CBHW081144280526

45787CB00007B/3219